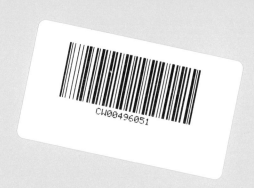
CW00496051

BOOZE
LESS

Rethinking
Drinking
for the
Sober & Curious

BOOZE
LESS

A GUIDED JOURNAL

By Millie Gooch

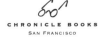

CHRONICLE BOOKS
SAN FRANCISCO

Copyright © 2024 by Millie Gooch.

All rights reserved. No part of this product may be reproduced in any form without written permission from the publisher.

ISBN 978-1-7972-3122-8

Manufactured in China.

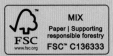

Design by Liz Li and Vanessa Dina.

10 9 8 7 6 5 4 3 2 1

While I have approached the content in this journal with care, consultation, and thought, it is not, and should never be, a replacement for proper medical or psychological help. If you or a loved one are struggling with alcohol, please be sure to seek a medical professional's help and consult the resources at the back of the journal. Everything I have included in this journal comes from my experience and the experiences of those in my community, but it may not be your experience.

For some people, quitting drinking can be dangerous, and a detox of this kind should be carried out under medical supervision. Please consult your primary care provider before making drastic changes to your drinking habits.

Chronicle books and gifts are available at special quantity discounts to corporations, professional associations, literacy programs, and other organizations. For details and discount information, please contact our premiums department at corporatesales@chroniclebooks.com or at 1-800-759-0190.

Chronicle Books LLC
680 Second Street
San Francisco, California 94107
www.chroniclebooks.com

For Mum, Dad, and James.
Would change the surname, wouldn't change you.

CONTENTS

INTRODUCTION

Oh, hey there.

My name is **Millie,**
and I have a loud
and busy brain.

After making it through more than three decades on this strange planet, I've found that only a handful of things make my hectic little head feel a smidge less chaotic, the most notable two being writing and drinking alcohol.

I started writing as soon as I could, well, write and spent most of my childhood shunning outdoor play for producing poems, diary entries, and short stories. My love for writing led me to pursue a degree in English Literature and Language and then a career in journalism.

I started drinking when I was around eighteen, which is relatively late in some cultures, but I made sure to make up for lost time. My drinking led me to several bar jobs, many dark headspaces while hungover, and that one time I woke up at the very end of a train line.

In my early twenties, drinking took over writing as my favorite pastime/coping mechanism, and those years were mostly spent either drunk, hungover, riddled with anxiety . . . or a combination of all three. There were good times, of course, but over the years, those became less and less frequent. At the grand young age of twenty-six, after years of binge drinking and blackouts, I decided to put my mental health first and embark on a journey of sobriety.

It has been six years since I started that journey. Since then, I've founded a supportive community for sober and sober curious women, written a book on how to drink less and live more, and created the journal you're holding right now.

Although I didn't realize it at the beginning, writing about my experience of sobriety in real time was one of my best tools for

- **Processing all the big feelings I faced when I stopped drinking**

- **Understanding the patterns behind my destructive drinking**

- **Recognizing patterns of behavior in general**

- **Holding myself accountable**

- **Releasing the fears I had about what would happen if I stopped drinking**

I've always been passionate about the power of the written word when trying to share ideas with others. And these days, I'm just as much an advocate for writing as a way to communicate with *ourselves*. By putting pen to paper, I can untangle the messy feelings in my mind—and put them back in my brain with a little more structure and order.

But anyway, this journal is not about me (check out the first book for that); this journal is about you. Gorgeous, wonderful you.

If you're reading this, it means you'd like to explore your relationship with alcohol. Well, you've come to the right place.

So, what should you expect? First off, this journal is designed for everyone. Yes, everyone. Whether you are looking to banish booze from your life forever, have been sober for a while but want a refresh as to why, or merely want to take a break and take stock, this journal will be your right-hand companion.

The best way to use this journal is chronologically, as we'll be moving through the stages of sober curiosity, from becoming a mindful drinker to creating a life you love without alcohol. But I'm not here to judge, so if you'd rather dip in and out, be my guest!

And while we're talking about judgment, I just want you to know this: There is none. This journal isn't aiming to convert you to forever sobriety; it is simply a space for you to get curious and understand your relationship with alcohol. (Though if you do decide to bin the booze for good, that's wonderful too.)

I won't keep you much longer, but here are a few final things to note:

- **There's no rush to complete all the prompts, so take as long as you need. You can take a break at any point; there is no timeline.**

- **The more you write, the more you'll get out of this journal. In this context less is not more, so dive deep and embellish to your heart's content.**

- **Honesty is the best policy. No one is going to read this journal (unless you ask them to), so tell the truth, the whole truth, and nothing but the truth!**

- **Try to stay open-minded and be kind to yourself. Alcohol consumption is a tricky, challenging, and often confronting subject, so the prompts might require you to address things you've never considered. Push yourself gently and with a healthy dose of compassion, and consider consulting a professional, like a therapist or counselor.**

- **Lastly, I'm not judging you, so you better not judge yourself. Life gets busy. If you forget about this journal for a few weeks, skip a few prompts, or cross things out, no worries. Just pick it back up and crack on. We're aiming for mindfulness, not perfection.**

Now let's get boozeless!

becoming a

MINDFUL

drinker

THERE'S A POPULAR CONCEPT IN THE SOBER SPHERE KNOWN AS MINDFUL DRINKING, AND WHILE IT MIGHT SOUND A BIT NEBULOUS, DRINKING MINDFULLY SIMPLY MEANS BECOMING MORE IN TUNE WITH YOUR BODY AND BRAIN WHEN IT COMES TO ALCOHOL CONSUMPTION. BECOMING AWARE OF YOUR DRINKING HABITS, UNDERSTANDING YOUR RELATIONSHIP WITH ALCOHOL, AND MAKING MORE INTENTIONAL DECISIONS REGARDING DRINKING ARE ALL WAYS TO CULTIVATE A MINDFUL DRINKER'S MINDSET.

Really, mindful drinking is interchangeable with the notion of being *sober curious*—it just sounds fancier!

So, this begs the question: What *isn't* mindful drinking? Some surefire signs of mind*less* drinking are

- Drinking out of habit or as part of a routine
- Frequently ordering your next drink before finishing the one that you already have
- Drinking because it's easier than having to explain why you don't want to
- Knocking back shots (even though you find them repulsive)
- Drinking just because everyone else is and you don't want to feel left out
- Regularly blacking out or suffering from hangover anxiety because of your drinking

If any of these prompted an enthusiastic nod (or perhaps a subdued one if you're currently battling a hangover), then you're in the right place because this section is all about getting mindful and understanding your relationship with alcohol. After all, you can't change something that you don't fully understand.

The exercises in this section have all been designed to help you learn more about alcohol, uncover the reasons why you drink, and illuminate what may be holding you back from truly embracing a hangover-free lifestyle.

LET'S GET STARTED!

THE FIZZY POP QUIZ

You know that classic dream where you're taking an exam that you didn't even study for? Well, brace yourself because that scenario just got real— although thankfully, this time you're not in your birthday suit.

1. What is alcohol made from? _____

2. There are different types of alcohol.
   Which kind is used in alcoholic beverages? _____

3. **True or false:** Alcohol affects men and women
   differently. _____

4. Every alcoholic drink has an ABV percentage on
   the label. What does ABV stand for? _____

5. How many different cancers has alcohol
   consumption been linked to? _____

6. What organ in the body primarily processes
   alcohol? _____

WHY UNITS MATTER

You may have heard someone say that you shouldn't consume more than a certain number of "drinks" per week. But it's important to observe that not all drinks are created equal when it comes to their alcohol content and the impact they have on the body. Instead, I encourage you to think about alcohol in terms of "units" (the more common term in the UK) rather than in drinks (or glasses of wine/beer).

Do you know what a unit of alcohol looks like? We're about to find out! Guess how many units each of these drinks contains:

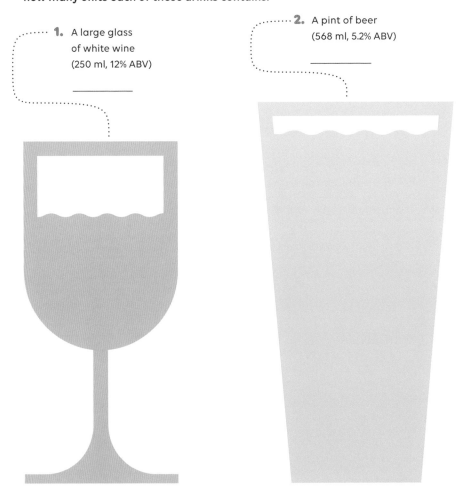

1. A large glass
of white wine
(250 ml, 12% ABV)

_____

2. A pint of beer
(568 ml, 5.2% ABV)

_____

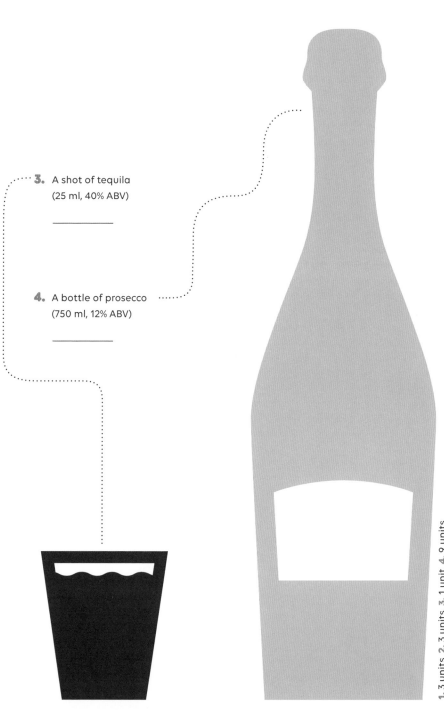

3. A shot of tequila
(25 ml, 40% ABV)

_____

4. A bottle of prosecco
(750 ml, 12% ABV)

_____

1. 3 units 2. 3 units 3. 1 unit 4. 9 units

DID YOU PASS?

If you spectacularly botched both quizzes—perfect, that's exactly what was supposed to happen.

So, why set you up for failure? Well, even though the world boasts over two billion alcohol drinkers, most of us have no idea what it is that we're regularly ingesting or how it affects us both in the short and long terms. Likewise, most of us have no idea just how much we're drinking either.

While it can be a little overwhelming, possibly even frustrating, to learn this information, gaining this knowledge will empower you to make decisions about your alcohol consumption.

KNOWLEDGE IS POWER

It was a few months after I quit drinking, when I had less brain fog and more mental clarity, that I really started to reflect on my own dynamic with alcohol. Akin to the ending of a romantic relationship, I found myself constantly trying to make sense of where it had all gone wrong. How had alcohol turned from something I sporadically used for fun to something that had become an essential part of how I navigated and made sense of the world? How had it gone from being something I could happily turn down to one of the main informants of both my pleasure and pain? It was only when I stepped back soberly that I could see just how messy and complicated my relationship with alcohol had become.

Obsessed with trying to rationalize my toxic entanglement with booze, I started learning about the very substance itself. I wolfed down books, inhaled podcasts, and binged on every documentary I could find, learning about the elusive liquid that had kept me in a chokehold for most of the previous decade.

I learned that alcohol was considered by some scientists to be the most harmful drug in the world—that had it been discovered today, it would likely not be legal. I learned that you don't really forget what happened on a night out, but that alcohol's effect on memory processing means that some things never make it from your short-term memory to your long-term memory. Alcohol essentially turns you into a human version of *Finding Nemo*'s Dory (with less swimming and more slurring). I learned that when you black out, you can be dancing, singing, or chatting, and the people around you may have no idea that you're in a bad state. I learned that hangover anxiety happens partly because you can't remember your night but also because of an actual chemical process. I learned that some people are more predisposed to addiction, that some people find abstinence easier than moderation, and that the alcohol industry is heavily involved in decisions around alcohol policy. I learned that even a month off alcohol could improve sleep and start to repair liver damage and that some of my favorite actors and musicians had been teetotalers for years.

There are many tools that help me navigate the world as a nondrinker—most of which I plan to share in this journal—but I truly believe that knowledge is the most powerful one. The more facts about alcohol we hold in our arsenal, the better equipped we are to understand things like why and how it can make us feel *less than* and how subtle yet inescapable the symptoms of mindless drinking can be. Learning about alcohol, what it is, and how it affects our mind, body, and life means that we can make more informed decisions around how, when, and indeed *if* we consume it. Pursuing this knowledge is the first step in becoming a mindful drinker.

Now that we know a little more about booze—let's get into how it shows up in *your* life.

EMOTION POTIONS

A lot of us drink to *feel* something: more confident, less stressed, or more connected to the people around us. Fill out the emotion potion labels with the feelings you try to attain by drinking.

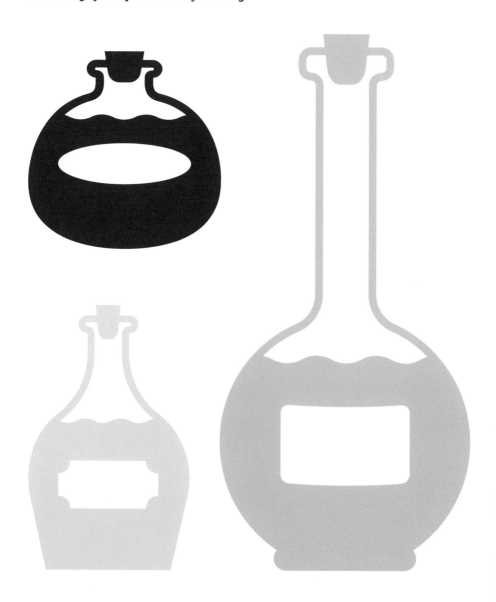

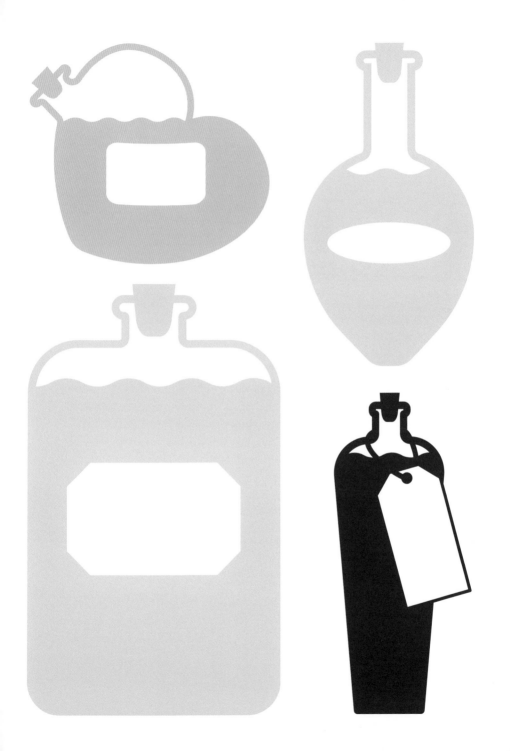

IDENTIFYING YOUR TRIGGERS

In the simplest terms, triggers are things that make you want to drink. They could be places (like certain bars), people (like certain friends), songs, TV shows, or even something as abstract as the weather.

Of course, you can never avoid triggers entirely, but being aware of the things that set you off is helpful so that you can put tools and strategies in place as preventative measures. It's also useful to think about *why* these things are such a strong catalyst, so that you can start to find some central themes to your drinking. A therapist or a counselor might be able to offer more insights into these triggers as well.

I've given you examples for each category that I've crowdsourced from the Sober Girl Society online community.

Using this list as a starting point, try to add as many triggers as you can.

Who is it?	Why do they trigger you?
Example 1: My boss	*They constantly put me down and make me feel like I'm not capable at my job. I think drinking alcohol after work helps me deal with those feelings and stops me from ruminating on their remarks.*
Example 2: My friend Jack	*He's made a few comments recently about how much more fun I am when I'm drinking, and now, I'm worried that he hates my company when I'm sober—so I always just end up drinking around him, just in case.*

Where?

Where is it?	Why does this place trigger you?
Example 1: My Mum's house	*My parents are divorced, but my Mum still lives in my childhood home. I find it hard being in that house, and I always just accept any drink she offers me—usually wine!*
Example 2: Weddings	*Going to other people's weddings makes me feel like I'm behind in my own life, so I just always end up getting drunk. I also think they're just long days, and drinking tops up my social battery.*

What is it?	Why does it trigger you?
Example 1: The sun	I think I associate sunny weather with having an Aperol Spritz. I'm not sure if summer would feel the same without it or if I would get FOMO.
Example 2: Cooking	I always have a glass of wine when I'm making pasta at home. It's part of the ritual, and I feel like I don't enjoy cooking without it!

When?

When is it?	Why does it trigger you?
Example 1: Sunday evenings	*I always get really stressed about going back to work on Mondays, so I feel like alcohol helps me wind down at the end of the weekend.*
Example 2: When I feel tired	*My emotions always feel really heightened when I'm tired, and I get very easily overwhelmed. I feel like drinking mellows me out when this happens.*

Who? Where? What? When?

Who/where/what/when is it?	Why does it trigger you?

USE THESE EXTRA PAGES FOR OVERSPILL!

35

Who/where/what/when is it?	Why does it trigger you?

Who/where/what/when is it?	Why does it trigger you?

Who/where/what/when is it?	Why does it trigger you?

Who/where/what/when is it?	Why does it trigger you?

Who/where/what/when is it?	Why does it trigger you?

Who/where/what/when is it?	Why does it trigger you?

BURN YOUR BELIEFS

A lot of us hang on to old beliefs that no longer serve us, and beliefs about alcohol are no exception. Maybe you believe that you'd never be able to go on a date without alcohol or that your friends wouldn't understand if you declined a drink. Perhaps you believe that you wouldn't be able to get on a dance floor without having had a few. Use this space to write down every belief you have about alcohol that could be preventing you from changing your relationship with it. Then, rip out the pages and burn them.

Disclaimer: I understand that for some, ripping pages out of a book and sacrificing them to the flames feels like a crime against the literary universe. So, if you'd rather do this on a separate piece of paper, you have my sympathetic understanding.

NOW RIP THEM OUT AND BURN THEM— SAFELY!

ME, ME, ME

They say that if you're not willing to give, then you shouldn't expect to receive. I don't know who "they" are, but since I'm about to ask you to deep-dive into your drinking and dish up some intimate details, I think it's only fair that I reciprocate with some reflections about my own consumption (including some of my own triggers, previous beliefs, and reasons for getting so hammered in the first place).

It starts with my brain, a place so chronically chaotic that I'd liken it to an airport on Christmas Eve, in which thousands of tiny passengers are having hundreds of tiny thoughts, and 90 percent of those thoughts are inane, impulsive, and irrational.

Aside from being asleep, the only time my mind felt a sense of serenity was while I was drinking. Known as *alcohol myopia*, booze has the ability to focus your concentration on immediate events and distract it from past or future events. For someone like me, who manages to stress about the past and the future simultaneously, alcohol can feel like the perfect escape—an easily accessible way to finally feel present and connected—at least for the first few drinks. After that, I was about as present as a shadow in the dark.

I spent most of my early twenties feeling deeply insecure and struggling with my mental health. I resented the way I looked; I hated that I always felt "too much" but also somehow not enough; and I struggled with anxiety, depression, and forever feeling "a little bit mental." From the outside, it wasn't obvious. To most people I was confident, bubbly, and the epitome of a twentysomething party girl. Temporarily, booze silenced my inner critic, lifted my spirits, and provided relief from the buzzing in my brain. But by using alcohol in such a way, drinking became so enmeshed with my personality that when I finally did stop, I wasn't sure where my hot-mess persona ended and the actual me started. Having relied on alcohol for expressing both confidence and personality, I hadn't bothered to create an identity of my own. Truthfully, I wasn't entirely sure who I was without alcohol. But more on that later!

In terms of my triggers, these included but were not limited to: the airport, festivals, pub gardens, watching episodes of *Sex and the City*, dating apps, bad dates, good dates, any dates, feeling anxious, feeling overwhelmed, and finally, the Friday free bar at work (because I'm convinced that anything tastes better when you don't have to pay for it).

If I was burning my beliefs, we'd probably have to start with the big one: that I'd be boring without booze. Having carefully crafted my entire personality around being an unrepentant hedonist, the idea that people might consider me safe, vanilla, and reliable gave me a feeling probably best described as "the ick." I also believed that no one would find me attractive if I didn't drink, my friends wouldn't want to hang out with me, I'd spend the rest of my life feeling socially awkward, and I'd never again feel the wild rush of living on the edge. I'm pleased to report that even after more than six years of not drinking, none of my beliefs ever materialized, and I promise, it's likely yours won't either.

SOBER STARS

Evaluating your drinking can sometimes be a lonely experience. Luckily, in the last few years many sober and sober curious celebrities and notable names have talked openly about their relationship with booze! When I first stopped drinking, I loved finding out that people who were doing amazing things in the world also didn't drink. In a weird way, it made me feel less alone. Use this space to add any celebrities (or even friends/family) you admire who don't drink or have a mindful approach to drinking.

under the

INFLUENCE

NOW THAT YOU'VE GAINED SOME INSIGHT INTO THE "WHY" OF YOUR DRINKING, IT'S TIME TO **LOOK AT THE IMPACT** ALCOHOL IS CURRENTLY HAVING ON YOU AND YOUR ABILITY TO LIVE THE **GREATEST LIFE POSSIBLE**. THE PROMPTS IN THIS SECTION HAVE BEEN LOVINGLY AND NONJUDGMENTALLY DESIGNED TO HELP YOU IDENTIFY THE PRESENT INFLUENCE DRINKING IS HAVING ON EVERYTHING IN YOUR LIFE, FROM YOUR FINANCES AND RELATIONSHIPS TO YOUR **PHYSICAL AND MENTAL WELL-BEING**.

Throughout this section, please try to remember that the impact of alcohol on an individual's life is a completely relative one. What might feel catastrophic to one person might not warrant a second thought from another. Some folks can write off the huge sums of money they spend on nights out as "pocket change." But for others, these splurges may send them spiraling further into already overwhelming debt. Likewise, hungover heart palpitations might be readily accepted as part and parcel of last night's fun by some; but if you're prone to health anxiety, the worry over bizarre physical symptoms could derail your entire week.

I also want you to be wary of (and ideally avoid) binary or cookie-cutter thinking, whether that means assuming problematic drinking always presents itself the same way in everyone or comparing your drinking patterns to those of your pals. The only thing that matters in this section is how you feel about *your* relationship with alcohol. No comparisons and no "shoulds." Personal relationships with alcohol are not one-size-fits-all.

Sorry, that sounded a little demanding. As a peace offering, would you like to come and play bingo with me?

HANGOVER BINGO

According to one study,* a hangover may encompass up to forty-seven symptoms! Cross out all the ones you've experienced, and if you get a full house . . . I'm glad you're here.

*Ruske Penning, Adele McKinney, and Joris C. Vester, "Alcohol Hangover Symptoms and Their Contribution to the Overall Hangover Severity," *Alcohol and Alcoholism* 43, no. 3 (2012), 248–252.

HANGOVER BINGO

FREE SPACE	Thirst	Drowsiness	Sleepiness	Headache	Dry mouth	Nausea
Weakness	Reduced alertness	Concentration problems	Apathy	Increased reaction time	Reduced appetite	Clumsiness
Agitation	Vertigo	Memory problems	Gastrointestinal complaints	Dizziness	Stomach pain	Tremor
Balance problems	Restlessness	Shivering	Fatigue	Sweating	Disorientation	Audio sensitivity
Photo sensitivity	Blunted affect (difficulty feeling or displaying emotions)	Muscle pain	Loss of taste	Regret	Confusion	Guilt
Gastritis	Impulsivity	Hot/cold flashes	Vomiting	Heart pounding	Depression	Palpitations
Tinnitus	Nystagmus (rapid, repetitive and/or uncontrolled eye movements)	Anger	Respiratory problems	Anxiety	Suicidal thoughts	FREE SPACE

AN ODE TO HANGOVERS

I wake up in the morning,
with a pounding in my head.

Then a wave of sickness hits me,
next, existential dread.

My memories are hazy,
I've got a sense of ick.

Do all my friends now hate me?
Did I call my boss a dick?

Where on earth's my bag,
my phone, keys, and ID?

How did I get home last night?
Oh god, I need to pee.

I find my phone, unlock it.
Two texts sent to my ex.

One says, "I still love you."
The other one's a hex.

I try to call my best friend,
no luck, perhaps she's mad?

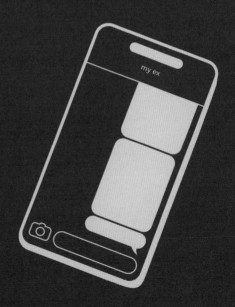

my ex

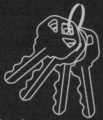

Now I'm starting to feel anxious,
and that quickly turns to sad.

I'm not sure how it happens,
how I take it just too far.

'Cause I always end up messy,
and stumbling out the bar.

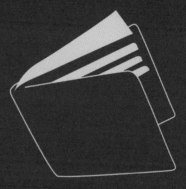

The guilt starts sinking in.
I soon get back in bed.

But the restless thoughts are whirring,
constant racing in my head.

Half of me is starving.
Half of me can't eat.

Half insists we shake it off,
then half admits defeat.

I spend the whole day crying,
and start to wonder when,

I'll really mean it when I say,
"I'm never drinking again!"

BOOZY BALLADS

Come on, Shakespeare. Now it's your turn to wax lyrically! Whether you want to compose a haiku, pen a limerick, or craft a sonnet, use this space to get honest with how you really feel about drinking and hangovers.

THE WHEEL OF DRINKING

The wheel of life is a common tool used in coaching practices. Usually, this exercise requires you to shade in (or color) each of the designated segments, reflecting how satisfied you are with that part of your life.

For example, if you've just won the lottery, you might shade your finance portion all the way up to a ten, or if you've just been dumped by the love of your life, perhaps your romantic relationships segment will remain firmly unshaded at zero. But we're going down a slightly different route.

The wheel of life is now the wheel of drinking. For each slice of the pie, you will assess the current impact that alcohol is having on that part of your life. For example, if alcohol is causing you to shake with hangover anxiety every Sunday morning, maybe you'd shade more segments on the mental health portion. Perhaps if you only booze once a month and your job has remained unimpacted, leave the career portion blank. In this wheel, rather than shading how satisfied you are with each section, you're shading to see how much of a negative impact alcohol is having on that area of your life.

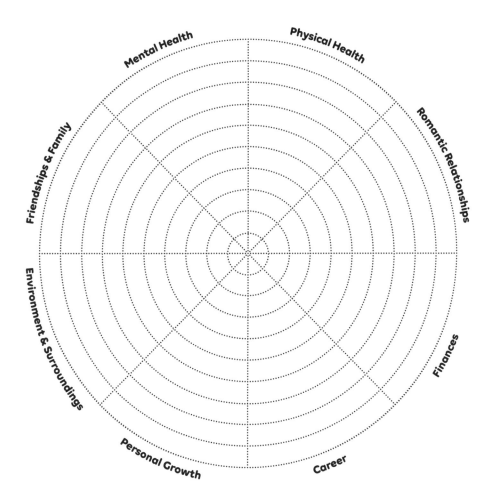

NOTE: Although alcohol production can have a negative impact on our lovely blue planet, the environment label in this exercise is more about your immediate surroundings. Do hangovers mean you never get around to cleaning the bathroom? Is your bin overflowing with empty bottles and your sofa covered with beer stains?

Now that you've numerically contextualized the impact of alcohol on each key part of your life, it's time to provide real-world examples. For each segment, please describe a situation in which alcohol has had an undesired impact.

Mental health:

_____

_____

_____

_____

_____

_____

_____

_____

_____

_____

_____

_____

_____

_____

_____

_____

_____

_____

_____

_____

Physical health:

_____

_____

_____

_____

_____

_____

_____

_____

_____

_____

_____

_____

_____

_____

_____

_____

_____

_____

_____

_____

_____

_____

_____

_____

Romantic relationships:

Finances:

Career:

Personal growth:

Environment & surroundings:

Friendships & family:

THE TROUBLE WITH "NOT THAT BAD"

When I first stopped drinking, a number of people told me I was "not that bad" and that I didn't have a "drinking problem." It immediately struck me as an odd, and somewhat insensitive, reaction. At the end of my drinking career, I was regularly blacking out and putting myself in dangerous situations, and my mental health was at an all-time low—and yet I didn't *quite* meet their criteria for "bad" or a "problem."

I thought a lot about what else needed to happen to me, or what I needed to look like to the world, in order for people to put their invisible approval stamp on my application to the sober club. I thought about the people who *were* considered "that bad"—the Hollywood stereotype of a troubled starlet checking into rehab—and wondered why I was being compared to them. As it turned out, the world thought I needed to tick all the boxes instead of just most of them.

It soon became clear to me that "drinking problems" are viewed by society in a much different light than other problems we may encounter. In my book, *The Sober Girl Society Handbook*, I compared house fires, of all things, to problematic drinking. Most people, upon seeing a house fire, would attempt to put it out instantly because, well, wouldn't it be rather peculiar to wait until your home is fully ablaze before deciding to spring into action? Whereas with problematic drinking, we merely wait, and wait, and wait some more. (Often, by the time we finally spring into action, it's already spiraled out of control.)

Even if we compare alcohol to other substances, the same conclusion can be drawn. Generally, people who give up smoking cigarettes usually do so as a preventative measure. I've never heard someone declare they've given up smoking only to be met with "But you don't have a problem!" or "You're not that bad!" Drinking is the exception, not the rule. It is something you are supposed to persevere with until hitting some arbitrary threshold of "bad." Then, and only then, can you say you have a "problem" and have your application to the sober club accepted.

The idea of "not that bad" perpetuates the misconception that there is a clearly defined line between "normal drinking" and alcohol dependency when in reality, *alcohol use disorder* (the preferred scientific term) exists on a far-ranging spectrum. By constantly telling the millions of drinkers who are struggling with alcohol consumption (but perhaps don't medically qualify as alcohol dependent) that their habits aren't "that bad," we're discouraging any kind of self-reflection or introspection—and are ultimately preventing a whole host of people from reevaluating their relationships with alcohol.

INSTEAD OF ASKING YOURSELF, "DO I HAVE A DRINKING PROBLEM?" TRY ASKING, "IS DRINKING CREATING PROBLEMS FOR ME?"

INDIRECT IMPACTS OF INTOXICATION

When it comes to our mental health, alcohol can affect us in two ways: directly and indirectly. Directly might mean feeling anxious because of the chemical effect of alcohol; while indirectly could mean being so hungover that you can't bear to speak to anyone for the entire weekend, and so you wind up canceling plans at the last minute, abandoning the social connection your mental health would have greatly benefited from.

We're used to focusing on the direct ways that alcohol impacts us, but this is your space to think about all the indirect effects. Maybe you've skipped a coffee date or brunch plans with a friend one too many times, or maybe you've stayed inside the house all day long on a gorgeous sunny day— whatever it is, there's no shame here! Trust me; it's a worthy and telling exploration.

HOW DOES YOUR GARDEN NOT GROW?

There's a trick practiced in the gardening world: If you want to stop plants from getting too tall, spray an alcohol mixture on the plant's leaves. In the case of foliage, alcohol *literally* hinders growth.

Channel your inner shrubbery and think about all the ways in which alcohol might be stunting your progress and holding you back from reaching your full potential! Use the blank spaces on the pots to jot down your findings.

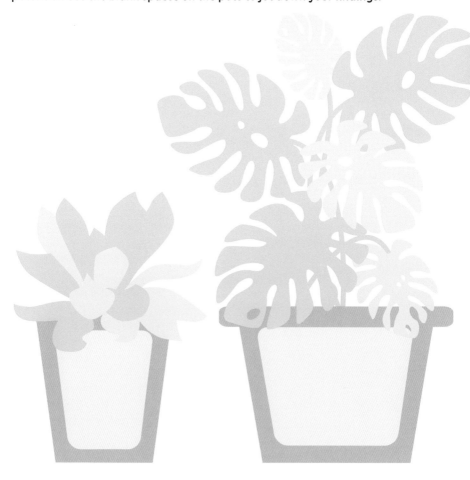

the
BOOZE
BREAKUP

ALTHOUGH SLIGHTLY **EMBARRASSING** TO ADMIT (BUT ISN'T THAT WHAT WE'RE HERE FOR?), I'VE BEEN THROUGH MY FAIR SHARE OF BOTH BREAKUPS AND RELATIONSHIP SABBATICALS. SO I THINK I HAVE ENOUGH CREDIBILITY TO SAY THAT **BOOZE BREAKUPS** BOAST MANY SIMILARITIES TO **ROMANTIC BREAKUPS**.

From learning who you are without your sidekick to understanding that "good times" don't necessarily equate to "good for you," a booze-based breakup requires all the same tools and grieving time of an amorous split.

This section is all about helping you navigate the idea of a booze break, get comfortable with the idea of saying "see-ya" to the sauce, and learning how to be a little more independent.

I know, I know—breakups can produce all sorts of sad and scary emotions. But don't worry; you're not alone. We're going to do this one together. And if we are going to do this,

WE'RE GOING TO NEED SOME MUSIC!

HEARTBREAK ANTHEMS

You might not be following the traditional breakup routine of downing shots and drunk-dialing your ex, but that doesn't mean you can't blast out the empowering breakup tunes. Use these discs to create your booze-free playlist, and once you've finished, maybe hit Play while we crack on with this section!

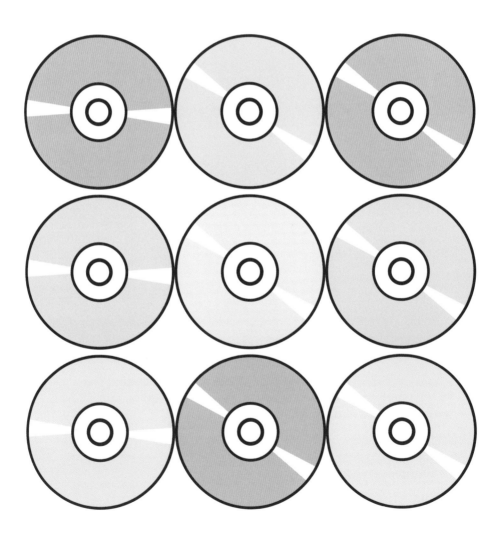

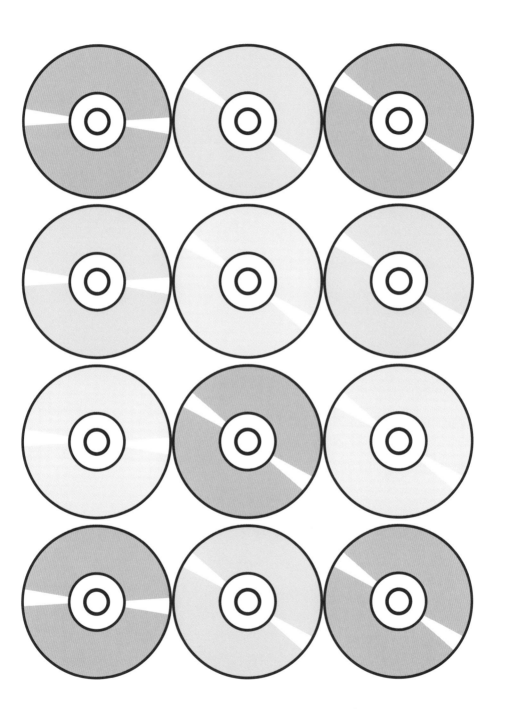

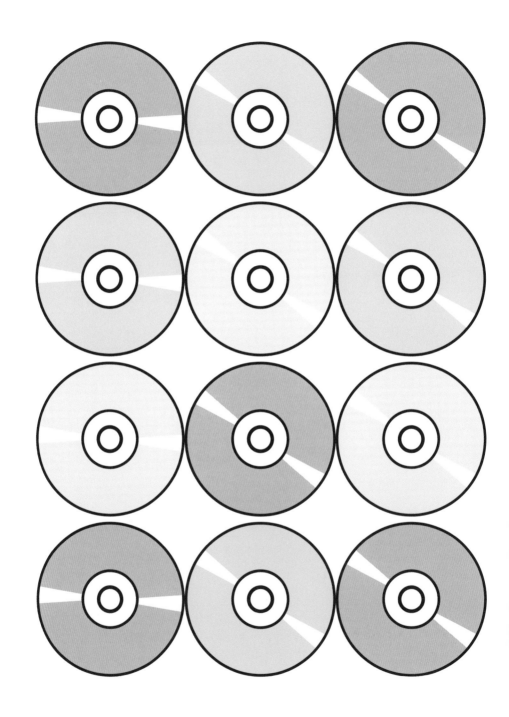

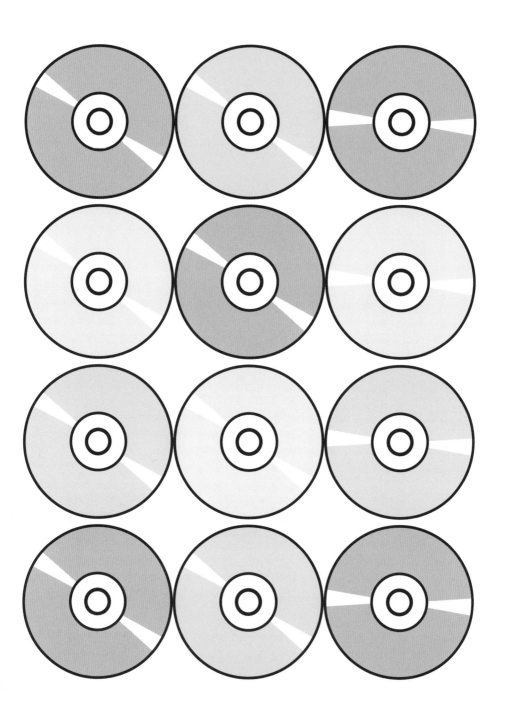

COOLING IT OFF

Not everyone wants to break up with booze forever, and that's totally okay! Maybe you're simply craving a bit of space or needing some time apart to reevaluate your relationship with it.

Whether you're pressing pause or ditching drinking for good, here are a few of my tried-and-true pointers for surviving those tricky initial stages.

Block them on social media. It's hard to stop thinking about something that constantly pops up when you're innocently scrolling on your favorite app. Unfollow any pages that are focused on drinking, like meme accounts or club nights. If you want to go one step further, you can use ad blockers on some social media platforms so that you're not inundated with alcohol marketing.

Go "no contact." To work out what you really want out of your relationship with alcohol, you need to spend some proper time apart. Even if you don't intend to say bye to booze for good, having at least 30 days away (though I recommend 90) from each other can provide you with enough space to get mindful about your relationship and envision how you might want it to look going forward.

Make sure you're in a good headspace when you see them. I've disregarded most relationship advice I've been given over the years, so if you're anything like me and decide to completely ignore the first two points, I understand. But at the very least, promise me that you'll be in a good headspace when you do decide to have contact with booze. Drinking when you're feeling down is likely to bring out the worst in you, often causing more harm than good.

Surround yourself with the right people. The main thing that has gotten me though every breakup is other people, especially supportive and loving friends whose sole concern is seeing me be happy. Isolation and loneliness can be a big trigger for unhealthy drinking habits, so choose to spend your time with people who you know will uplift you and back what you're doing.

Do things you wouldn't have done before. When you start gaining back your independence, it's the perfect time to start doing things you might have neglected during a relationship. Pick up discarded hobbies, start therapy, meet up with friends you haven't seen in a while, or finally get into that TV series you've been meaning to watch!

FILLING YOUR TIME

When something or someone exits our life, it can often leave us with a lot of extra time on our hands. A booze break is no exception.

Fill in this clock with all the things you want to use your newfound time for!

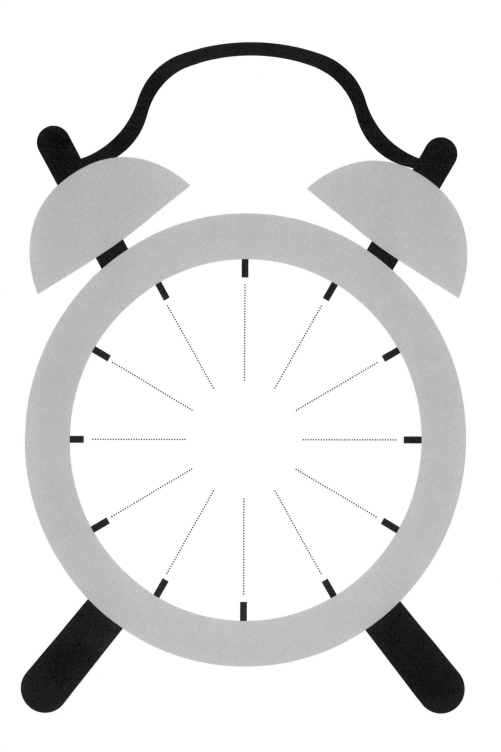

MAKING NEW MEMORIES

Now is the perfect time to break any negative associations you have with boozy things of the past by creating new, sober experiences.

Use this space to think about any places or experiences that might have been dampened, or even ruined, by drinking, which you would like to revisit in a more positive and present way. As you write, think about the following questions:

- What was the experience?

- How was it affected by alcohol?

- How would you like to change/revisit it with a sober lens?

RED FLAGS

After a breakup, we can often forgive the worst parts of a relationship and even go so far as to romanticize them. Use the red flags to point out booze's bad bits and why you're leaving it behind—refer to this list often!

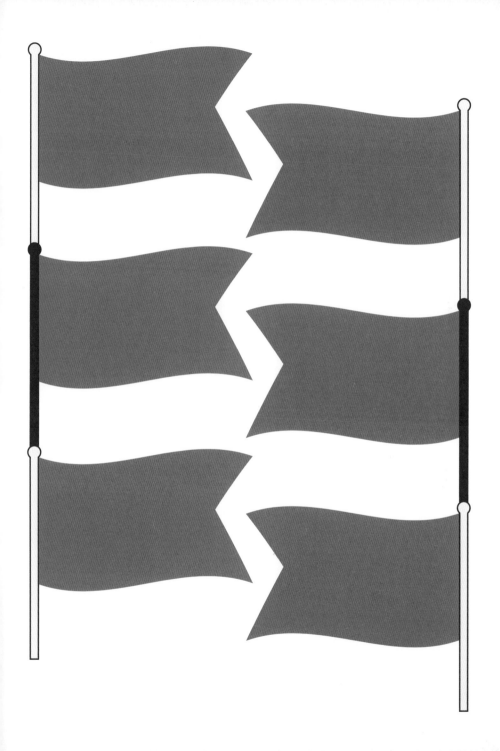

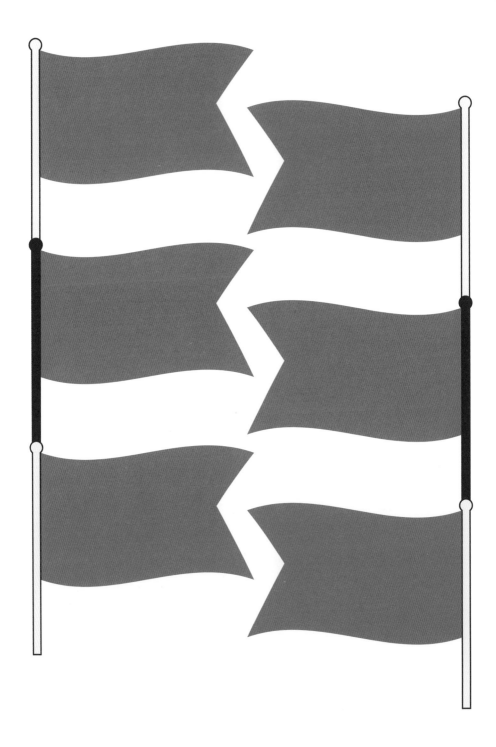

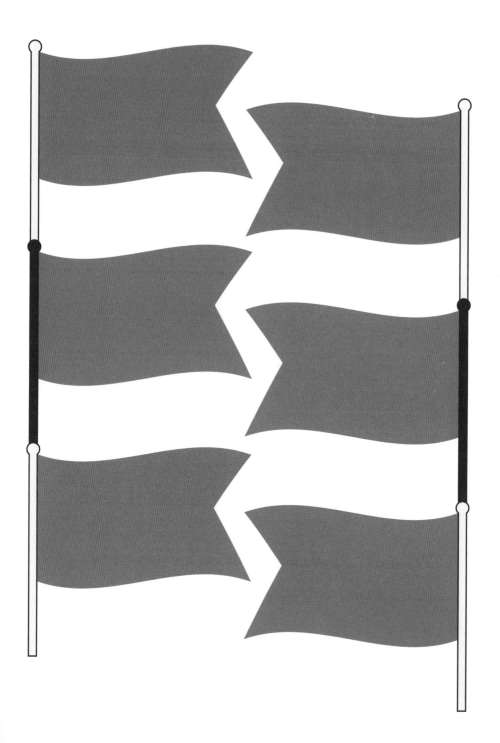

WHAT ARE THE PROS?

One of the oldest forms of journaling is the classic pros and cons list, historically rolled out when deciding whether or not one should be heading toward Splitsville. Your red flags from the previous page have served as your cons. Now, why not see if you can find some pros to alcohol?

This exercise may seem counterintuitive, but if you find pros (and no judgment if you do), I hope this will further enlighten your relationship with alcohol. And if you don't, the blank page in front of you should be just as illuminating!

PROS

THE FALLING-OUT-OF-LOVE LETTER

When it comes to any breakup, closure is important. In fact, I've written many letters to ex-partners (even if I haven't sent them) and always found the practice quite cathartic. So, use the space below to write a goodbye (or see you later) letter to alcohol and get everything off your chest!

YES, I KNOW IT FEELS AWKWARD, SO DON'T WORRY—I'LL GO FIRST!

Dear Alcohol,

How did we get here, eh? For many years of my life, you were someone I could always rely on for a good time, and we really did have a lot of fun together, didn't we? In so many ways, you made me the woman I am, or maybe you made me a woman I wasn't but one that I liked being at the time. You made me confident, sociable, and frankly, very chatty. However, I can't be sure if that was your doing because it's been a while since I last saw you, and now, I'm all those things and more. Maybe those things were in me all along—maybe I just relied on you too much? I never trusted that I was good enough without you.

I don't know when it all stopped being fun. I just know that at one point, things changed. The nights used to end in laughter, but they soon started ending in tears. I didn't always want to hang out with you by the end of our relationship, but I felt like I needed to, like I didn't know how to dance, talk, or exist in social settings without you.

Eventually, you became duplicitous: One version of you hushed my insecurities and negative thoughts, and another version encouraged them. On one hand, you assured me that I wasn't unlovable, that I belonged. On the other, during every "morning after," it was a different story. Because of you, I believed the worst about myself: that my friends all hated me, that everyone thought I was an embarrassment, that it would be better if I wasn't here. Worst of all, sometimes your influence made me do things that felt so out of character, so far removed from the person I really wanted to be. I'm not saying it's all your fault—I am taking some responsibility here—but let's face it: You were designed to make me depend on you eventually.

It wasn't always extreme. Sometimes you just made me feel a little low and that wasn't always that terrible. It's just that by the end of it all, the bad outweighed the good, the balance tipped, and eventually, I knew I had to let you go.

Anyway, it's been over six years since we've had any contact, and I can honestly say that without you, I have learned more about the world and how to show up in it than I ever did when you were part of my life. I've been forced to put myself in scary situations, step out of my comfort zone, and trust that I can get through anything. And I have.

I have learned to forgive, learned to forget, and come to the realization that perhaps if things hadn't ended so badly between us, I never would have found myself. For that, I am eternally grateful.

All my love,
Millie x

DEAR ALCOHOL . . .

Okay, now it's your turn!

the art of
SOBER
SOCIALIZING

WHETHER YOU'RE ON A BREAK WITH BOOZE OR IT'S MORE OF A WE-ARE-NEVER-EVER-GETTING-BACK-TOGETHER SITUATION, HEARTBREAK HIBER-NATION CAN'T GO ON FOREVER. IT'S OFFICIALLY TIME TO LEARN HOW TO SOCIALIZE—SOBER!

Socializing can be scary even at the best of times, especially if you're on the introverted side or neurodivergent, but doing it without an alcoholic beverage? Well, the thought is more than enough to send most people back into a destructive drinking cycle faster than you can say "happy hour." Not you, though—because luckily, you're in good hands.

Over the last six-plus years I've been to weddings, festivals, raves, concerts, networking events, first dates, mate dates, dinner dates, parties, clubs, and even a gin distillery—all without the aid of liquid courage to see me through.

ALL THIS IS TO SAY, YES, IT'S POSSIBLE!

ONCE UPON A
SOBER TIME . . .

Reflect on the last time you really enjoyed yourself or felt happy without alcohol. What were you doing? Who were you with? What made it so good? Feel free to embellish!

BOOZELESS BOUNDARIES

I know that *boundaries* has become a bit of a buzzword in recent years, but that's for good reason. Creating them around your drinking decisions can help you navigate the famously challenging early stages of sobriety. Boundaries also don't need to be extreme or worded in a specific way. For me, they looked like:

- "I'm more than happy give you a lift home if you don't mind leaving when I am ready to go."
- "I'm not getting involved in buying rounds of drinks. It's not because I'm being stingy, but there are only so many Diet Cokes one sober person can consume in an evening!"

Everyone's boundaries are different. Use this space to come up with five of your own that you might want to have on hand.

Remember, boundaries are about us creating protection around our own needs and limits. They're not about trying to control the behavior of others!

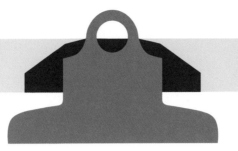

1.

2.

3.

4.

5.

THE JOY OF MISSING OUT

If you really think about it, sobriety is a little transactional. You give up things, and you get other things in return. In my opinion, better things. I find by focusing on what you're gaining from not drinking rather than what you're giving up, you can hone in on the positives.

While you might be familiar with FOMO (the fear of missing out), you might not be familiar with JOMO (the joy of missing out). JOMO is all about embracing the art of "no," of turning things down and filling that space with a heap of other things.

For example, you might feel FOMO through not drinking at parties, but in exchange, you might experience JOMO when meeting new people whom you connect with over that very subject.

So, you're going to donate ten FOMOs, and in return, you're going to give yourself ten JOMOs. Got it?

I'd like to swap this FOMO...

_____
_____
_____
_____
_____

For this JOMO...

_____
_____
_____
_____
_____

I'd like to swap this FOMO...

_____
_____
_____
_____
_____

For this JOMO...

_____
_____
_____
_____
_____

I'd like to swap this FOMO...

_____
_____
_____
_____
_____

For this JOMO...

_____
_____
_____
_____
_____

I'd like to swap this FOMO...

_____
_____
_____
_____
_____

For this JOMO...

_____
_____
_____
_____
_____

I'd like to swap this FOMO...

_____

_____

_____

_____

_____

_____

For this JOMO...

_____

_____

_____

_____

_____

_____

I'd like to swap this FOMO...

_____

_____

_____

_____

_____

_____

For this JOMO...

_____

_____

_____

_____

_____

_____

I'd like to swap this FOMO...

_____

_____

_____

_____

_____

_____

For this JOMO...

_____

_____

_____

_____

_____

_____

I'd like to swap this FOMO...   **For this JOMO...**

_____   _____
_____   _____
_____   _____
_____   _____
_____   _____
_____   _____
_____   _____

I'd like to swap this FOMO...   **For this JOMO...**

_____   _____
_____   _____
_____   _____
_____   _____
_____   _____
_____   _____
_____   _____

I'd like to swap this FOMO...   **For this JOMO...**

_____   _____
_____   _____
_____   _____
_____   _____
_____   _____
_____   _____
_____   _____

BEER PRESSURE

Until we have a massive societal shift, peer pressure around drinking is, sadly, inevitable. One thing I have found helpful is having a few rebuttals up my sleeve to use in response to unsolicited and judgmental commentary regarding my decision to abstain from alcohol.

You can use the talking heads below to think about how you could respond to what I've deemed the repeat offenders: some commonly experienced, unwarranted, and negative responses you may get regarding your choice not to drink. As you'll see, I usually opt for sarcasm, but whether you want to go the cheeky route, matter-of-fact route, or maybe even a dark-humor route is entirely up to you.

On the following page, you can fill in your own guesses of what you expect to hear when announcing your abstinence from alcohol!

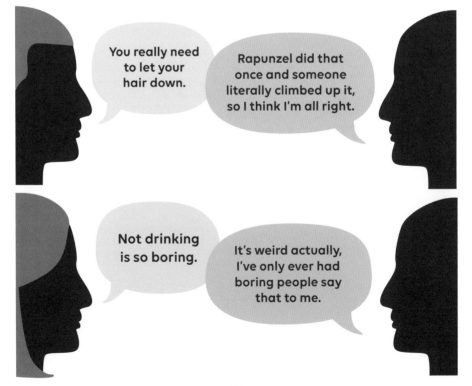

You really need to let your hair down.

Rapunzel did that once and someone literally climbed up it, so I think I'm all right.

Not drinking is so boring.

It's weird actually, I've only ever had boring people say that to me.

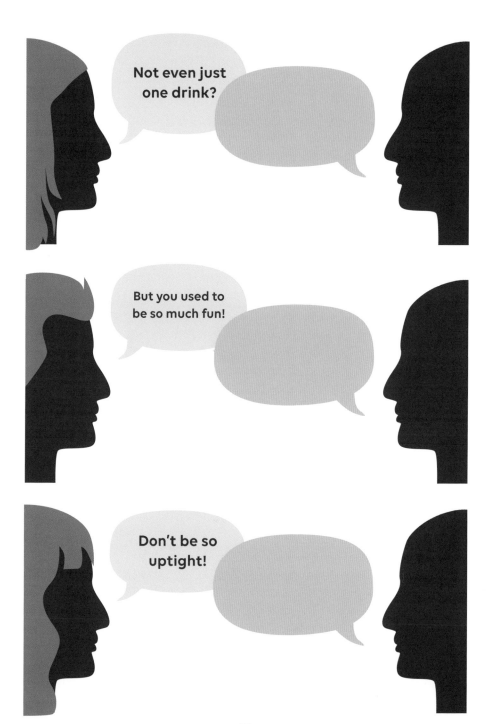

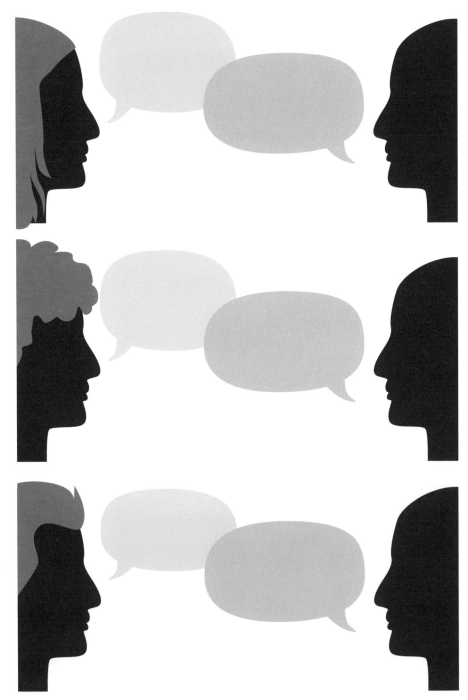

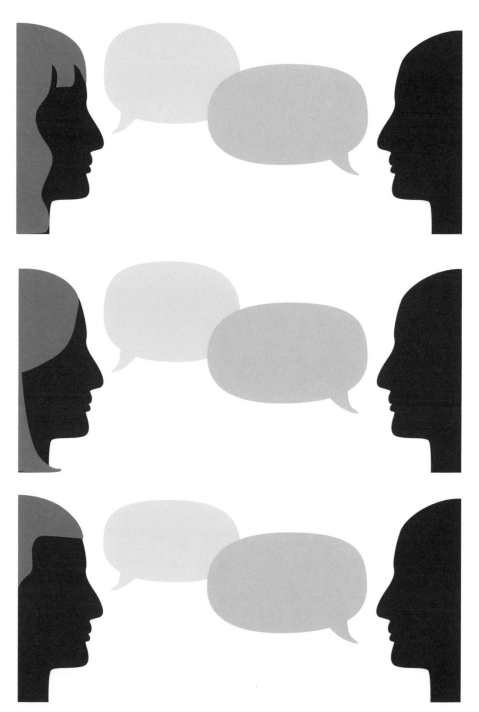

DRY COURAGE

If all my years of sober socializing have taught me one thing, it's that confidence is a skill, and while some people might like to think that confidence is something that you either possess or you don't, I truly believe that it's something you learn—just like any other ability or talent.

The problem is that many of us rely on alcohol (also known as liquid courage) for our confidence, so the thought of doing any social occasion without it is, quite rightly, terrifying. It's like the first time you get on a bike without training wheels or the first time you try to swim without floaties. You've been so used to having a safety net that without it you start thinking: What if I fall? What if I drown? What if I can't think of anything interesting to say and everyone thinks I'm a total embarrassment of a human?

But the truth is, at some point, cycling without the aid of extra wheels starts to be normal, swimming without inflatables attached to your arms becomes standard, and I promise you that one day, socializing without alcohol will feel completely doable. The reason? Practice, repetition, and self-discovery.

Confidence for sober socializing is something that you can absolutely learn and improve upon through repeatedly trying new things and seeing what form of socialization works best for you. Maybe you'll find that ditching the booze has made you an early bird who'd rather have a few close friends over for a cozy game night than go out dancing. Conversely, maybe you still love nightlife, and your new going-out routine will just take a bit of adjusting. One thing's for sure: You won't know until you try. Confidence for sober socializing is built by saying "yes" to things that might scare you at first, doing them, and realizing you can get through them, therefore feeling more prepared for the next thing, and repeating that process over and over and over again until infinity.

For example, I quickly realized that without alcohol, I tire earlier on nights out, but I usually still want to stick around for the late-night parties, so I decided that I should disco nap and down an iced coffee before going out if I know I will be out late. I also learned that during events where the focus was on drinking, such as a bottomless brunch or sitting in a pub, I'd often get bored easily. But I still wanted to see my friends, so I thought of games that we could play that would keep me engaged and be fun for all of us. Knowing that I have these tricks in my back pocket keeps me excited for social events and gives me confidence. I know I can attend and be an active participant without the crutch of alcohol.

Most importantly, it's good to remember that sober socializing is not one-size-fits-all, and that all of this will take time, as well as a little trial and error, so don't be disheartened if you're still nervous about it further down the line. It's completely natural to still feel nervous months or even years in because there will always be new events, new people, and new locations.

THE UNKNOWN IS WHAT SCARES US, BUT FACING IT IS THE ONLY WAY WE GROW!

THE CONFIDENCE JARS

A bit like a swear jar but nicer. Whether it's a date or dancing, every time you do something scary without alcohol, add it to the confidence jars to remind yourself of how brave you truly are!

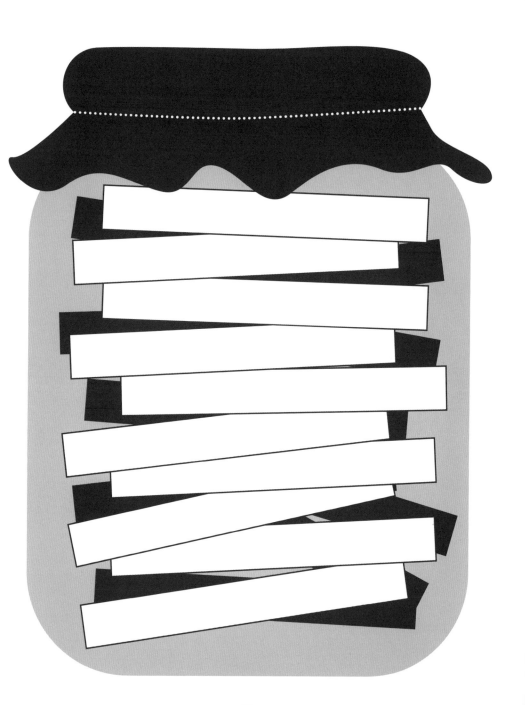

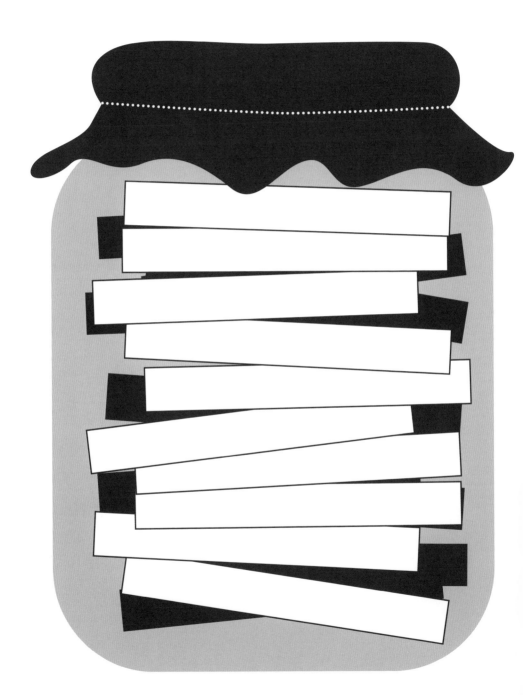

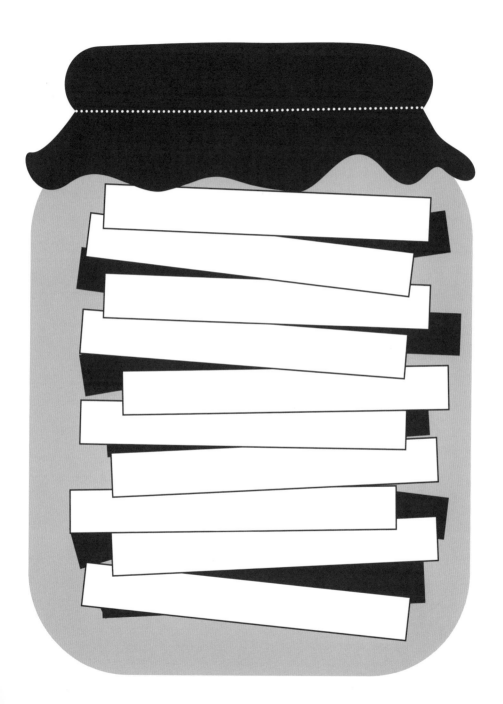

REDEFINING FUN

For a lot of us, fun = drinking. Which is all well and good until you put down the bottle and, as was the case for me, realize you have no idea what else you like doing for enjoyment. And while this is a daunting phase, it's also an incredibly exciting one that's full of potential. Drinking (and recovering from drinking) is incredibly time consuming. When you drink less, you get back a lot of time and disposable income (a night out isn't cheap). And when you realize there's a whole world of fun things to do that don't result in a headache, life can get pretty great.

NOT SURE WHERE TO START? TRY SOME OF THESE IDEAS.

Start a Pinterest board. Not just reserved for curating bathroom décor ideas, Pinterest boards are a great way to discover new interests, hobbies, recipes, and craft ideas. It is always the place I go to if I am lacking inspiration.

Reconnect with childhood hobbies. If you had activities or hobbies that you enjoyed doing when you were younger, consider bringing them back into your life. Not only are they a great way to connect with your inner child, but you might even find the whole thing quite healing. The key here is to challenge any internal narratives about what counts as "acceptable" for an adult. Miss playing on jungle gyms or in bouncy houses? There are adult versions now! Want to make daisy chains? What's stopping you?

Push back on the idea that everything must be productive. We live in a capitalist society, and while I'm not here to spout off about economics, it's important that I drum the idea into you that fun doesn't need to have a purpose, hobbies don't need to be monetized, and passion projects should always be about the process, not the end goal.

Join a group. While there are loads of sobriety groups, there are also plenty of other communities and hobby groups that don't revolve around alcohol. Whether you take up hiking or knitting, joining a group is also a great way to make new friends who are already practiced at sober socializing.

ONE HUNDRED HOBBIES

I polled the Sober Girl Society community to find out everyone's favorite nondrinking hobbies, activities, and new ways to make friends. Then I narrowed down the list to the top 100 contenders. Go through and check off all the ones that intrigue you, pique your curiosity, or give you a feeling of excitement!

○ 1. Acrobatics

○ 2. Amateur dramatics

○ 3. Archery

○ 4. Arts and crafts—resin, clay, etc.

○ 5. Badminton

○ 6. Baking

○ 7. Bird-watching

○ 8. Botany

○ 9. Boxing

○ 10. Bullet journaling

○ 11. Burlesque

○ 12. Calligraphy

○ 13. Camping

○ 14. Candle making

○ 15. Chess

○ 16. Circus skills

○ 17. Collecting—whatever you like!

○ 18. Coloring

○ 19. Concerts

○ 20. Cooking

- ○ 21. Crocheting
- ○ 22. Cross-stitching
- ○ 23. Cycling
- ○ 24. Dancing
- ○ 25. Diamond painting, not as expensive as it sounds!
- ○ 26. DJing/producing music
- ○ 27. Escape rooms
- ○ 28. Filmmaking
- ○ 29. Forest bathing
- ○ 30. Gaming
- ○ 31. Gardening
- ○ 32. Geocaching
- ○ 33. Ghost-hunting
- ○ 34. Glassblowing
- ○ 35. Going to a show (plays, musicals)
- ○ 36. Go-karting
- ○ 37. Golf
- ○ 38. Gymnastics
- ○ 39. Hiking
- ○ 40. Horseback riding
- ○ 41. Hula-hooping
- ○ 42. Ice/figure skating
- ○ 43. Improv theater
- ○ 44. Joining a sports team—basketball, soccer, etc.
- ○ 45. Kayaking
- ○ 46. Kickboxing
- ○ 47. Knitting
- ○ 48. Learning a foreign language

- ○ 49. Learning a musical instrument
- ○ 50. Learning sign language
- ○ 51. Learning to code
- ○ 52. LEGO®
- ○ 53. Magic
- ○ 54. Magnet fishing
- ○ 55. Makeup artistry
- ○ 56. Mocktail mixology
- ○ 57. Model building
- ○ 58. Museum visits
- ○ 59. Nail art
- ○ 60. Nonalcoholic wine/beer tasting—it's a thing!
- ○ 61. Orienteering

- ○ 62. Origami
- ○ 63. Opera
- ○ 64. Paddleboarding
- ○ 65. Paintball
- ○ 66. Painting
- ○ 67. Photography
- ○ 68. Pilates
- ○ 69. Podcasting
- ○ 70. Poetry readings
- ○ 71. Pole-dancing classes
- ○ 72. Pottery making
- ○ 73. Pottery painting (not the same thing!)
- ○ 74. Puzzles

- ○ 75. Reading
- ○ 76. Record collecting
- ○ 77. Rock climbing
- ○ 78. Roller skating
- ○ 79. Running
- ○ 80. Scrapbooking
- ○ 81. Sewing
- ○ 82. Singing/choir
- ○ 83. Skiing
- ○ 84. Snowboarding
- ○ 85. Spotting—planes, trains, clouds
- ○ 86. Stand-up comedy
- ○ 87. Stargazing

- ○ 88. Surfing
- ○ 89. Swimming
- ○ 90. Tai-chi
- ○ 91. Tarot reading
- ○ 92. Tennis
- ○ 93. Theme parks
- ○ 94. Upcycling
- ○ 95. Volleyball
- ○ 96. Volunteering
- ○ 97. Weightlifting
- ○ 98. Writing
- ○ 99. Yoga
- ○ 100. Zumba

THE ULTIMATE SOBER PARTY

As we near the end of this section, I want you to think about what could happen if you not only stopped dreading the idea of sober socializing but actively started getting excited about it. So, time to put your party planner hat on. If you were throwing the ultimate sober party, what would it look like?

The drinks:

_____

_____

_____

_____

_____

_____

_____

_____

_____

The food:

_____

_____

_____

_____

_____

_____

_____

_____

_____

_____

The venue:

_____

_____

_____

_____

_____

_____

_____

The music:

_____

_____

_____

_____

_____

_____

The decorations:

_____

_____

_____

_____

_____

_____

The dress code:

_____

_____

_____

_____

_____

_____

_____

The entertainment:

_____

_____

_____

_____

_____

_____

_____

The guest list:

_____

_____

_____

_____

_____

_____

_____

creating a

BOOZE
LESS

life you love

WHEN I STOPPED DRINKING, I FOUND THAT EVERYONE'S ADVICE FOCUSED ON THE **ACTUAL PROCESS** OF GIVING UP ALCOHOL, AND ALBEIT HELPFUL, IT LEFT ME WONDERING, **"BUT WHAT'S NEXT?"** THIS SECTION HAS BEEN DESIGNED TO GET YOU THINKING, AND POSSIBLY EVEN EXCITED, ABOUT WHAT **YOUR FUTURE** COULD LOOK LIKE **WITHOUT ALCOHOL.**

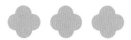

As this is our last section—cue tears—I've also left you with some final words of wisdom and resources that I hope will help you continue your quest of curiosity around mindful drinking.

NOW, LET'S GET ON WITH IT!

EASY LIKE
SUNDAY MORNING

I'm a big advocate of romanticizing everyday life, and when you stop drinking, idealizing the little things can help you fall in love with your sober or sober-ish existence. Use this space to describe your ultimate dreamy, hangover-free Sunday.

SOBER SHOPPING

If you're going to be saving money by drinking less or not at all, you might as well get excited about what you can spend the extra cash on. Make a wish list of a few items or experiences that you plan to splurge on with your booze-less savings!

1.

2.

3.

4.

5.

6.

7.

8.

9.

10.

11.

12.

13.

14.

15.

16.

17.

18.

19.

20.

21.

22.

23.

24.

25.

26.

27.

28.

29.

30.

AND . . . RELAX

So many of us use alcohol as a stress reliever or to chill out, so if you want to reduce your intake, finding new ways to unwind is key. Whether it's taking up yoga or screaming into a pillow, fill in the bubbles with the ways in which you plan to practice self-care. These can be old favorites or new routines you're eager to try.

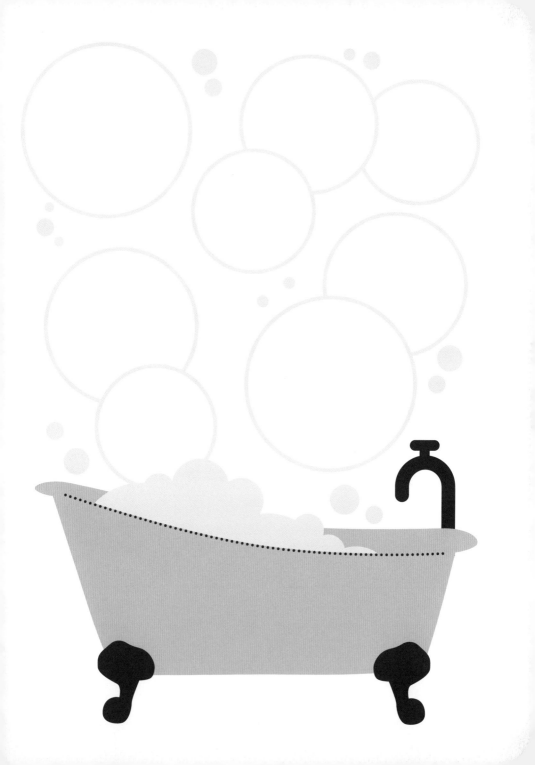

SOBER TOOLBOX

The concept of the *sober toolbox* is well known in sobriety circles. Essentially, a sober toolbox is your own personalized survival kit for when the cravings really hit. Your toolbox can contain physical items like herbal tea and your favorite blanket, but it can also include more conceptual things like podcasts or your best friend's phone number.

Use the blank spaces to fill your sober toolbox with everything that can help support you in your time of need.

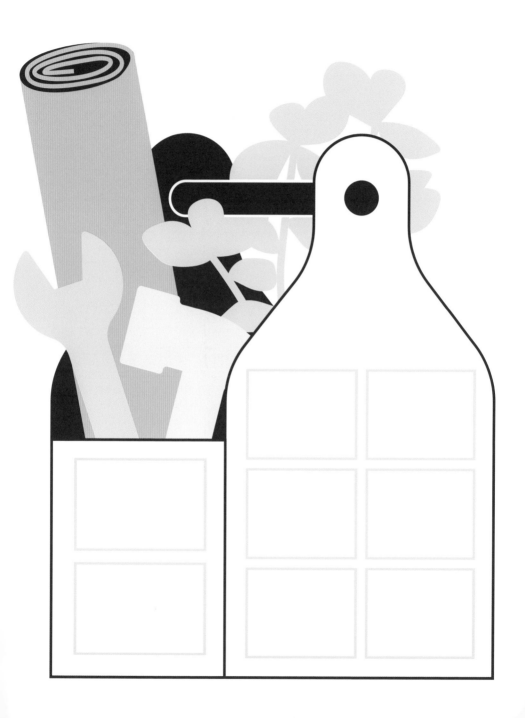

THE FIVE-YEAR PLAN

You know that annoying question you get asked in job interviews? "Where do you see yourself in five years?" Well, you're going to answer it. Twice.

First, you're going to reflect on where you see yourself in five years' time if you keep drinking. Then you'll picture your life in five years if you were to stop drinking (or practice mindful drinking). You can focus on all aspects of life that we've discussed thus far—financial, physical, or mental health; relationships; socialization; or your relationship to yourself. Nothing's off limits!

If I keep on drinking mindlessly, my life could look like . . .

If I stop or lessen my alcohol consumption, my life could look like . . .

THE PROMISE

We've reached the end of our prompts, so it's time to make a promise. Listen, we don't know each other too well, so let's be honest, a promise to me is kind of meaningless. *But* a promise to yourself? Now that's worth something.

Use this space to make a promise to yourself. It doesn't have to be a promise to stop drinking entirely; it can simply be a promise to start drinking more mindfully, or to take a thirty-day break every six months, or to try to stop worrying about what people think of your sober curiosity.

Dear me,

I promise . . .

_____

_____

_____

_____

_____

_____

_____

_____

_____

_____

_____

_____

_____

_____

_____

_____

_____

_____

_____

_____

_____

_____

_____

_____

_____

_____

_____

_____

_____

_____

_____

_____

_____

_____

_____

_____

_____

_____

Love,

A FINAL NOTE

I knew I needed to stop drinking way before I finally took the leap. For a long time, I ignored the little voice in my head that told me this—drowned out the noise of it with parties, pre-drinking, and poor decision-making. The little voice always knew what was best for me; I just wasn't ready to hear it.

Like I have said, this journal isn't here to recruit and convert you into some sort of teetotalistic cult. I won't be judging you if you close this journal and feel the urge to reach for a glass of wine. But what I do want you to do is *listen to the voice*. Not my voice, not the voices of other people—yours, and especially the little voice. The one that says, "This doesn't feel quite right" or "Maybe there is more to it all than this."

If you can't concentrate on the little voice, or maybe the other voices are too loud, *write*. Not only is writing one of the easiest ways to understand your own mind, but it is also a great way to let the little voice speak, and for it to be well and truly heard.

There's a big world out there beyond booze, and I can't wait to hear about how you tackle it.

LOOK AFTER YOURSELF AND KEEP IN TOUCH—THIS IS A SEE YOU LATER, NOT A GOODBYE.

All my love,
Millie x

ACKNOWLEDGMENTS

It's fair to say that I wouldn't be even a tenth of the person I am without the people around me, so this one is for them.

For the Gooch Family, Brighton Babes, Taboo, The Three Musketeers, Tuesday Club, Sober Boat Crew, Virtual Club, Tequila Tuesday (all unimaginatively/ironically named WhatsApp groups). Plus, Heather, who has managed to escape being added to any recent group chats.

For Lucy Gibson, who deserved a thank-you in the first book but didn't get one because I quite literally couldn't think straight. I once told her that if I organized a meetup, nobody would turn up—so she organized one to prove me wrong.

For Shaun, who was always there, no matter the circumstance. For angel Gaynor, too.

For Molly, who quite literally keeps the lights on at Sober Girl Society HQ, doing it with absolute kindness along the way.

For Team TBH, Verity, Seran and Lucy. Couldn't ask for better supporters, life organizers, or therapists.

For my actual therapist, Heidi, and David for all the pep talks.

For everyone at Chronicle, especially my editor, Alex Galou, who made me more excited about this project than I thought I even could be.

If I've learned anything about sobriety, it's that you need people who cheer you on, say nice things behind your back, and listen to the same problems repeatedly like it's the very first time they've heard them.

I feel very lucky to have that.

RESOURCES

BOOKS

The Sober Girl Society Handbook, by Millie Gooch (sorry, not sorry!)

The Unexpected Joy of Being Sober, by Catherine Gray

Drink? The New Science of Alcohol and Your Health, by David Nutt

PODCASTS

They Think It's All Sober

Seltzer Squad

Sober Curious

BLOGS AND WEBSITES

Sober Girl Society
https://sobergirlsociety.com/

Girl & Tonic
https://girlandtonic.co.uk/

CHARITIES AND ORGANIZATIONS

United Kingdom:

Alcohol Change UK
https://alcoholchange.org.uk/

Adfam
https://adfam.org.uk/

National Association for Children of Addiction (NACoA)
https://nacoa.org.uk/

United States:

Substance Abuse and Mental Health Services Administration (SAMHSA)
https://www.samhsa.gov/

National Association for Children of Addiction (NACoA)
https://nacoa.org/

Photo by Emily Metcalfe

MILLIE GOOCH

is the founder of the Sober Girl Society and is one of the voices leading the sobriety movement in the UK. As a journalist, she has written for a range of publications and has been featured everywhere from *ELLE* and *Stylist* to the BBC and *British Vogue*. Her debut book, *The Sober Girl Society Handbook*, was released in January 2021, and in 2022, she received the Media Award from the Research Society on Alcoholism for her contributions in helping disseminate empirical research on alcohol and creating a safe space for people to explore alcohol-free living.